Work Therapy

Work Therapy

written by
Daniel Grippo

illustrated by
R.W. Alley

One Caring Place
Abbey Press

Published by One Caring Place
Abbey Press
St. Meinrad, Indiana 47577

Library of Congress Catalog Number
95-75533

ISBN 0-87029-276-5

Printed in the United States of America

Foreword

Work, at its best, means fulfillment, gratification, learning, growth, and reward. It's a way we express our individuality, exercise our unique strengths, leave a mark upon the world.

Work also produces anxiety, frustration, tension, tedium, and disappointment. Work—or its lack—can make us feel harried, ineffective, inadequate, unsuccessful.

If work is bringing you less satisfaction and more stress, or if your workday is more boredom than bliss, you may need *Work Therapy*.

This small guidebook suggests ways to enhance your work life, to discover—or rediscover—joy on the job, to endure and learn from the tough times, to determine when it's best to move on, and to survive job loss.

Given all the ways we work—for a company, for our families, for ourselves; in an office, in a factory, at home, outdoors; for money or not—we spend a sizable part of our lives working.

You deserve to make that time the most satisfying and worthwhile it can be. Let *Work Therapy* work for you!

1.

Work, like love, is a many-splendored thing. Look at the variety of work you see going on around you. Marvel at its diversity, the multitude of abilities it demands, the abundant benefits it brings.

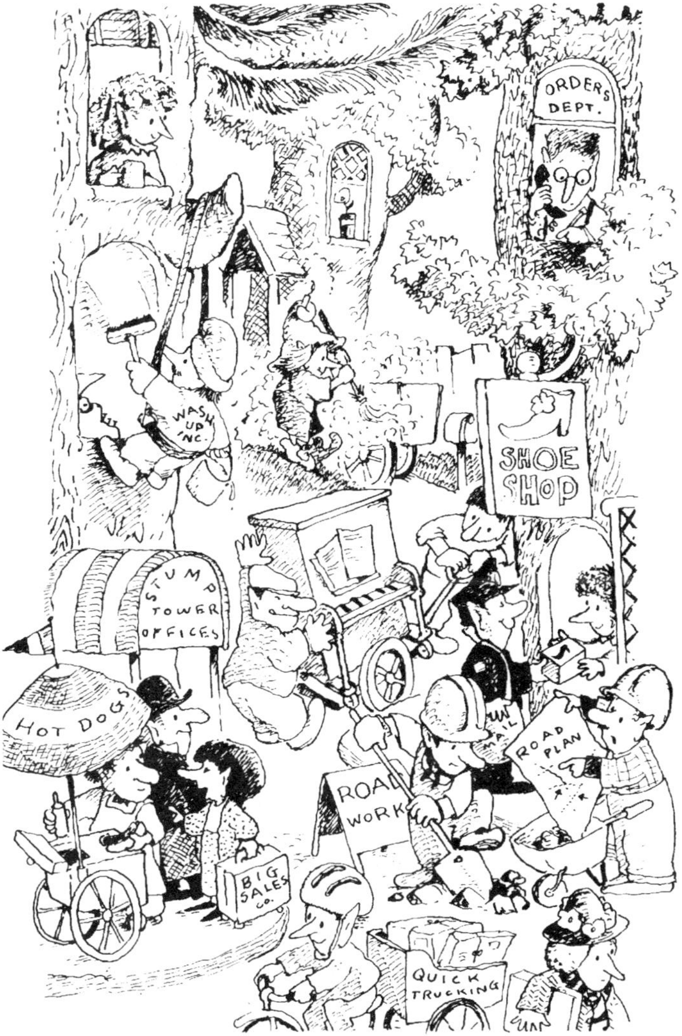

ORDERS DEPT.
WASH UP INC.
SHOE SHOP
STUMP TOWER OFFICES
HOT DOGS
MAIL
ROAD PLAN
ROAD WORK
BIG SALES CO.
QUICK TRUCKING

2.

All work has dignity. Any task, large or small, is important enough to be done carefully, thoroughly, mindfully. Take pride in your work—and in yourself for doing a good job.

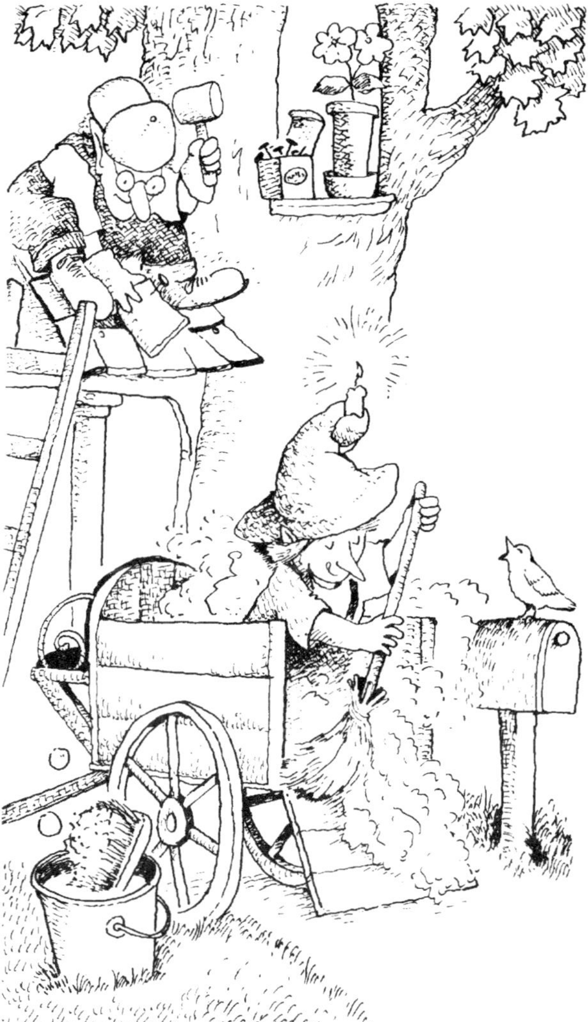

3.

Work doesn't have to be paid to be valuable. Notice how much of the really important work in life doesn't involve a paycheck.

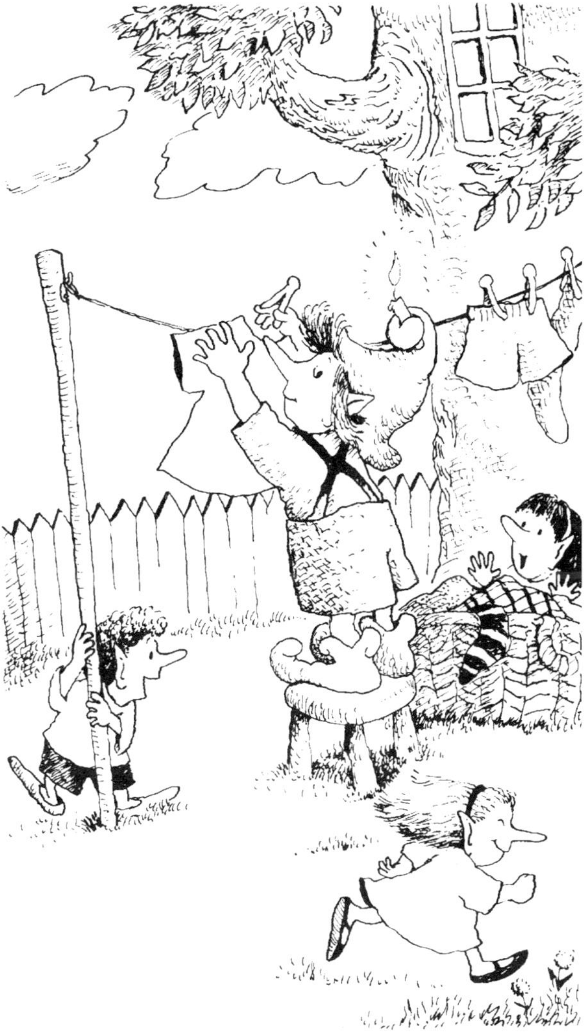

4.

All work can be creative. Your work is part of the ongoing creation of the world. See yourself as a co-creator with God.

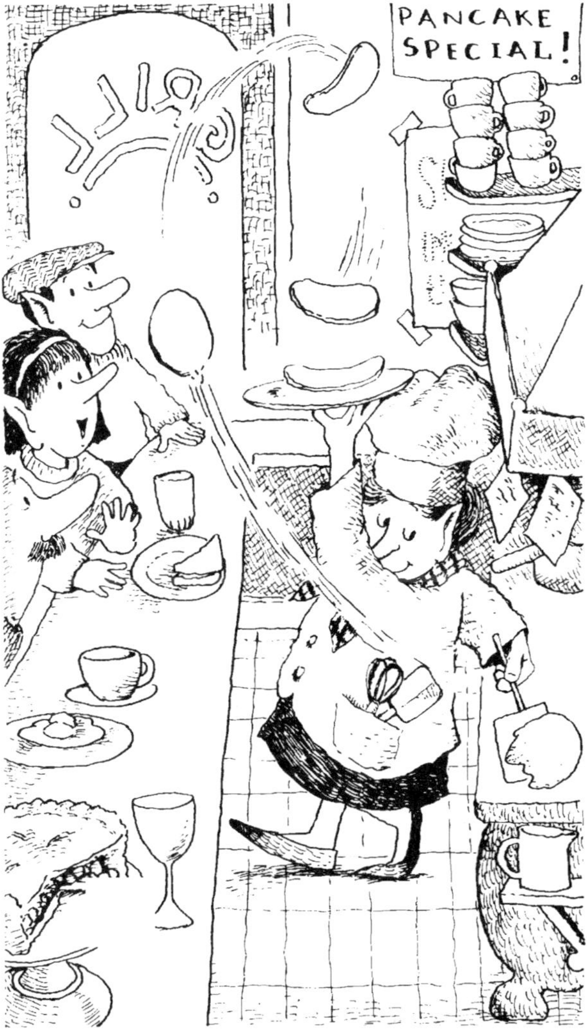
PANCAKE
SPECIAL!

5.

All work should preserve and be in harmony with creation. Find ways to save, economize, and recycle. Be a good steward.

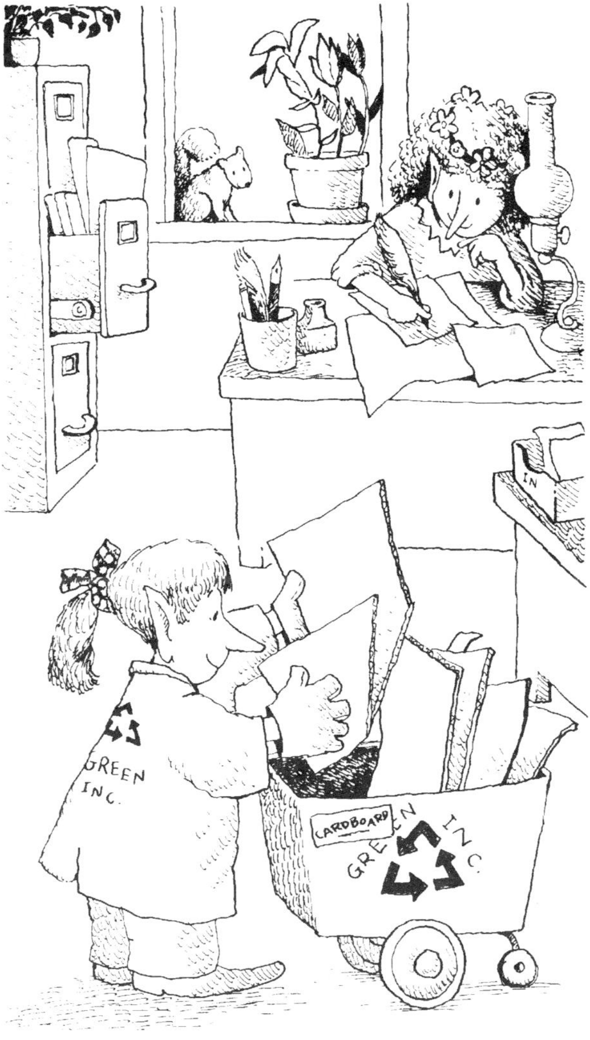
IN
GREEN INC.
CARDBOARD
GREEN INC.

6.

Cherish those moments of deep satisfaction in your work: arriving at a breakthrough idea, being part of a smoothly functioning team, discovering the answer to a vexing problem, feeling the good tiredness of a day well spent.

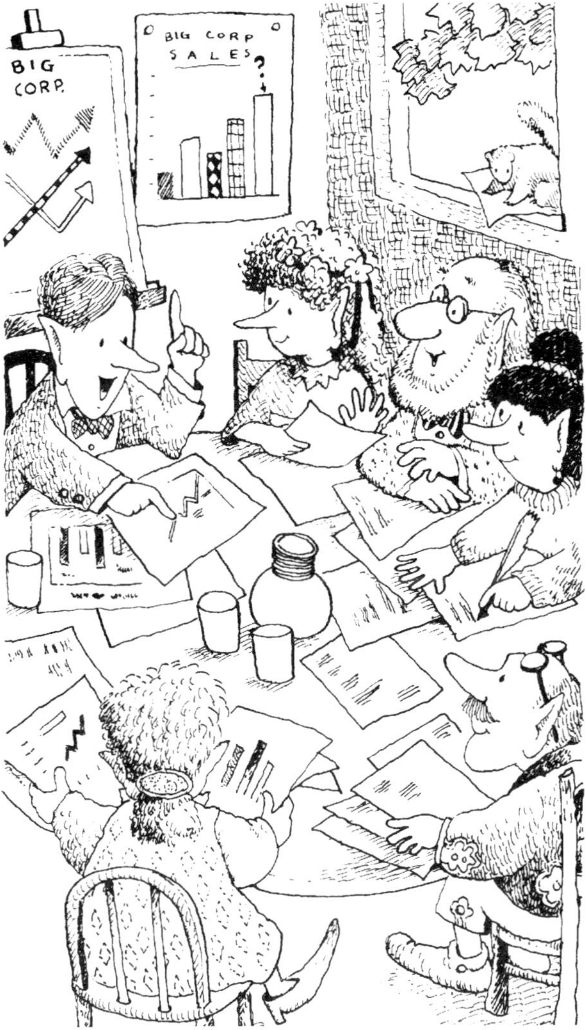
BIG
CORP.
BIG CORP
SALES

7.

Appreciate the hidden moments of joy in your workday: the warble of a robin outside a window, the scent of flowers on a desk, a funny story shared over lunch.

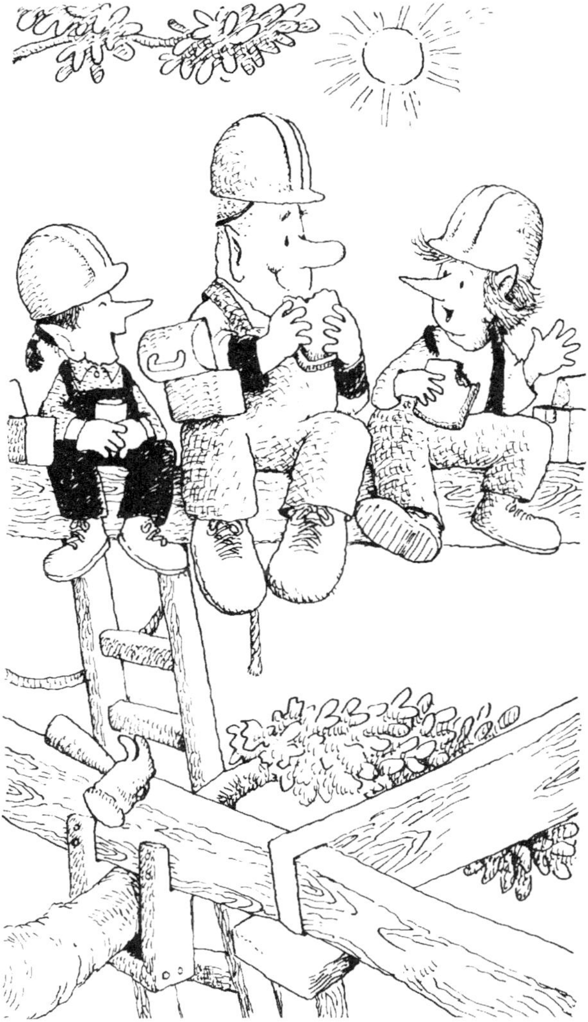

8.

When your work is stressful, take a momentary vacation. Stretch, look outside, walk around, take a beverage break, in your imagination surround yourself with what you love.

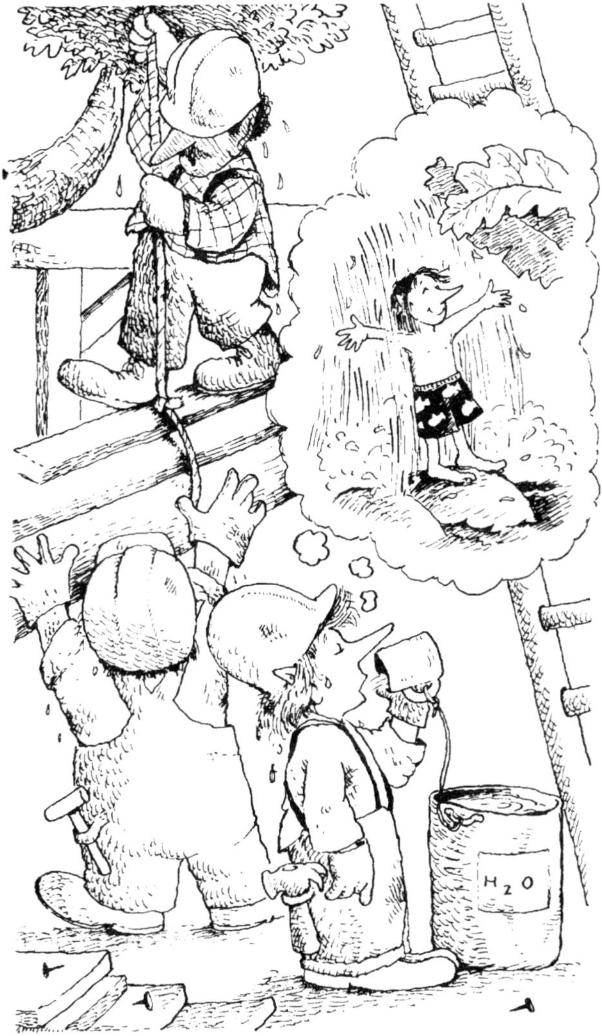
H2O

9.

Bring balance, rhythm, and variety to your work. Work with your hands as well as your head, with your imagination as well as your reason, alone as well as in groups.

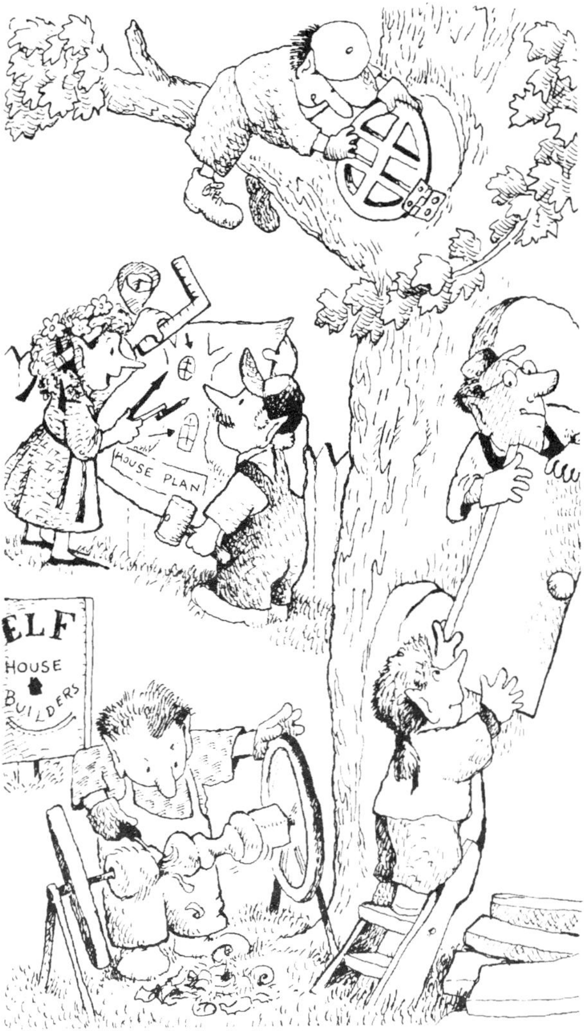
HOUSE PLAN
ELF
HOUSE
BUILDERS

10.

Enliven your workday by widening your work world. If you work inside all day, find ways to connect to the outside. If you work with or care for children, seek out contact with adults.

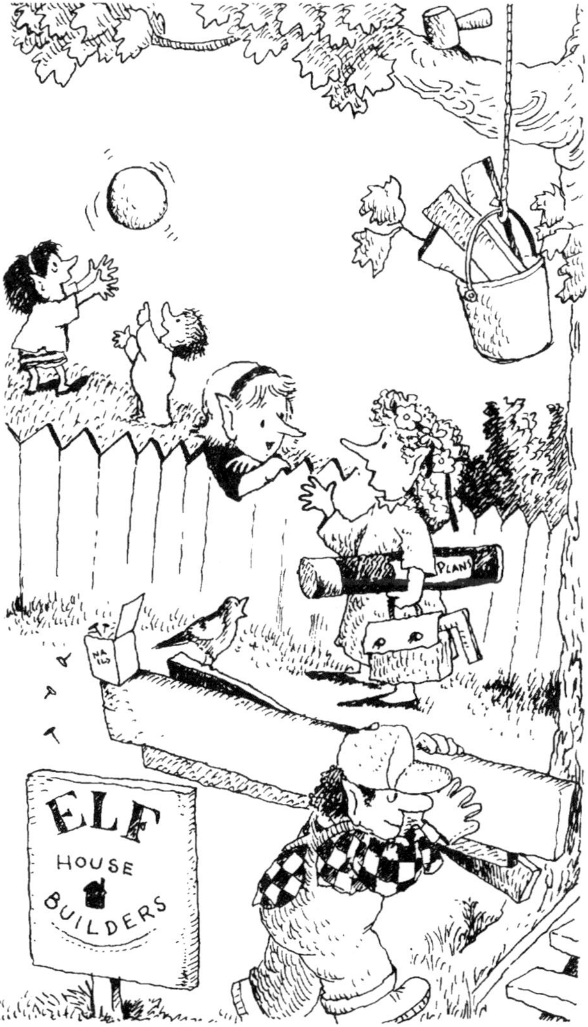
PLANS
ELF
HOUSE
BUILDERS

11.

When procrastination gets the better of you, imagine how good you'll feel when you've accomplished something. Remember that "Well begun is half done." Or, simply, "Do it."

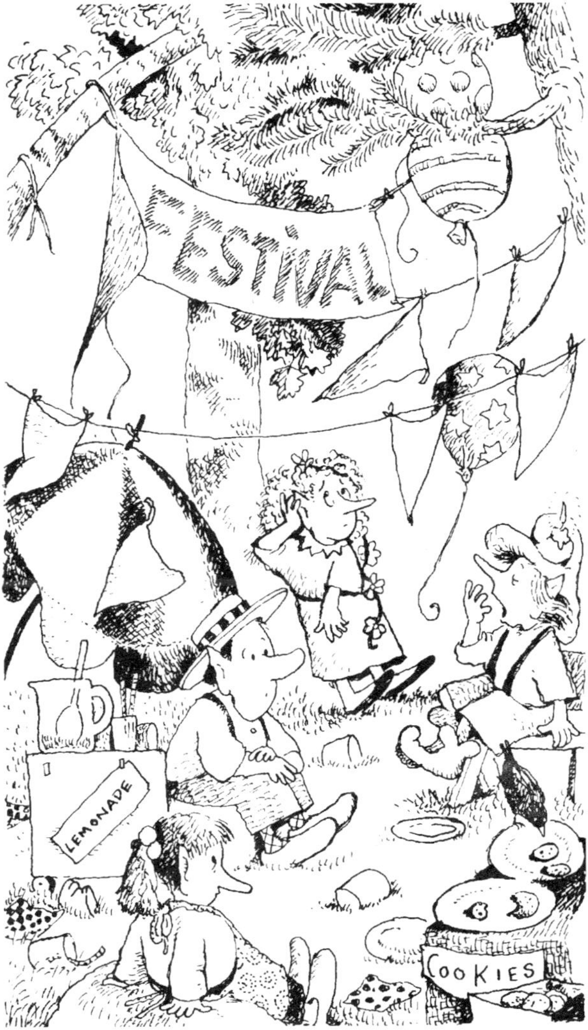

ESTIVAL
LEMONADE
COOKIES

12.

Don't try to do everything at once. When you're feeling overwhelmed, break a complex task into its smaller components. Decide what's most important and do it first.

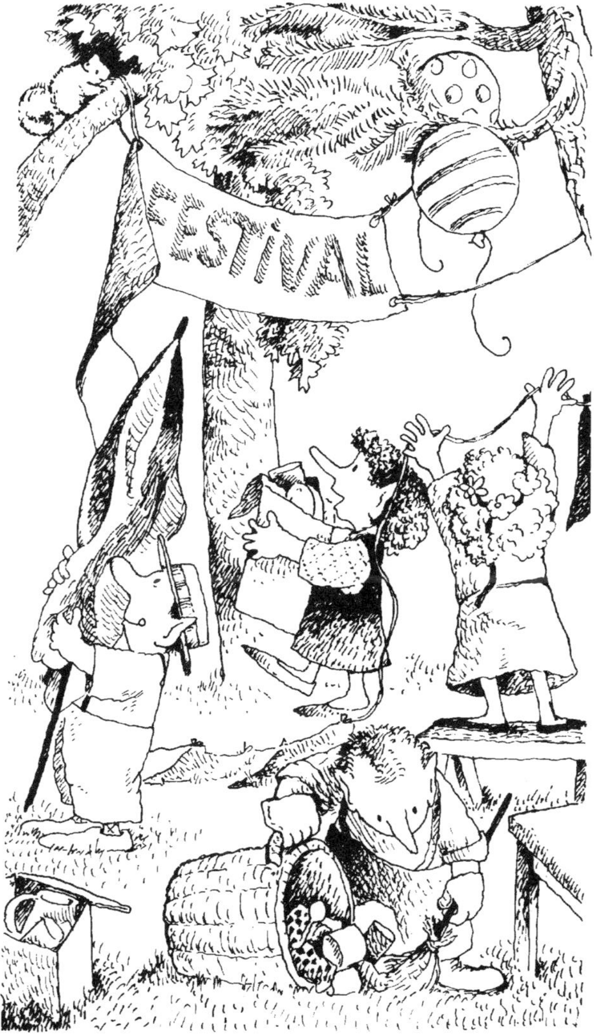
FESTIVAL

13.

Know the difference between being efficient and being effective. Efficiency is doing things right. Effectiveness is doing the right things. Both are important; don't sacrifice effectiveness for efficiency.

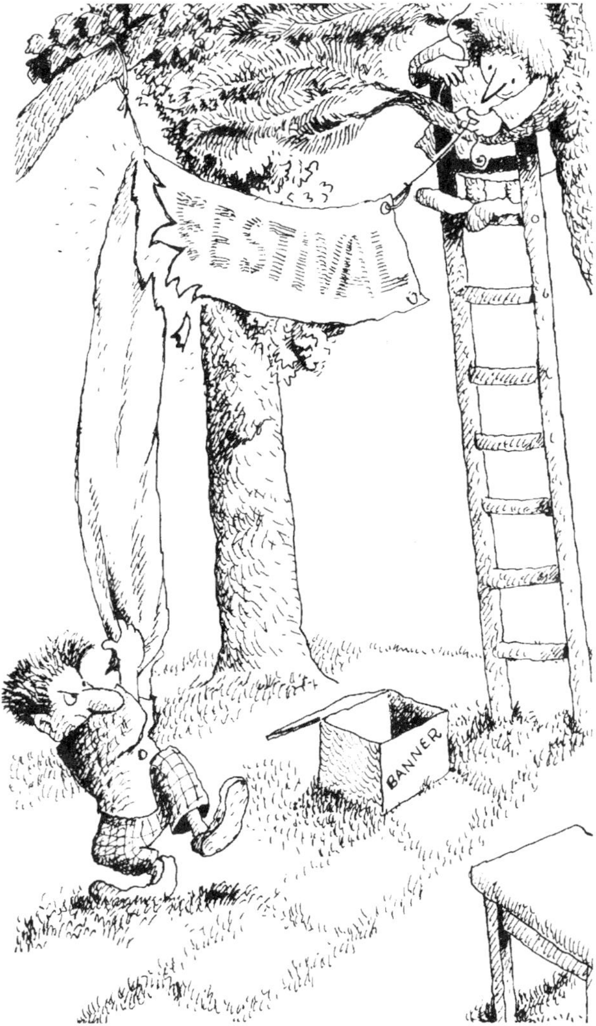
ESTIVAL
BANNER

14.

Set achievable goals and then recognize when you've reached each one. Take time to reward yourself and appreciate all you've accomplished, without worrying about all you have yet to do.

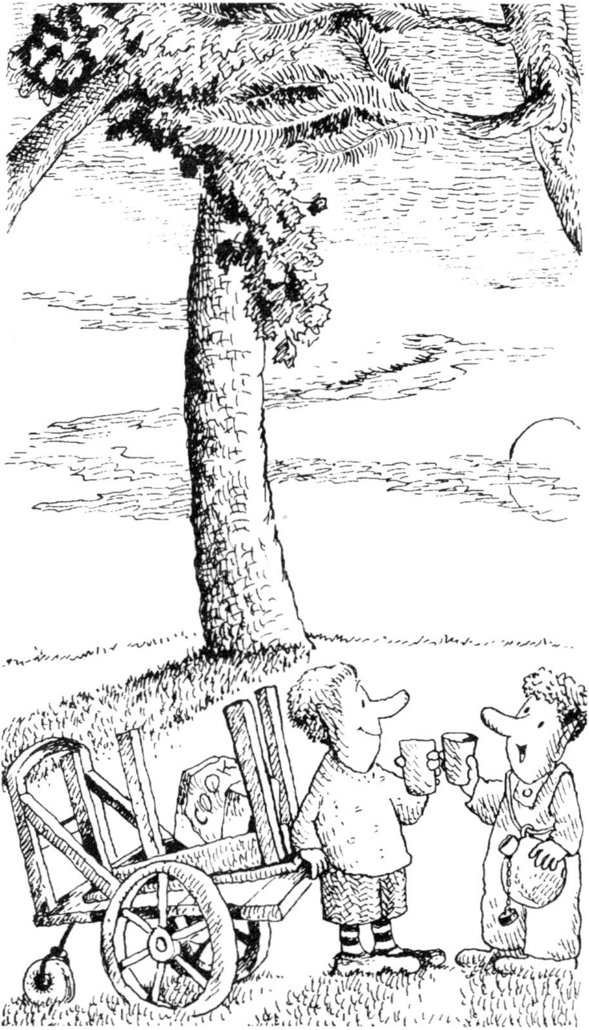

15.

Personalize your work space to create an environment that uplifts and pleases you. Photos of loved ones, artwork, plants, and favorite quotations can make a space your own.

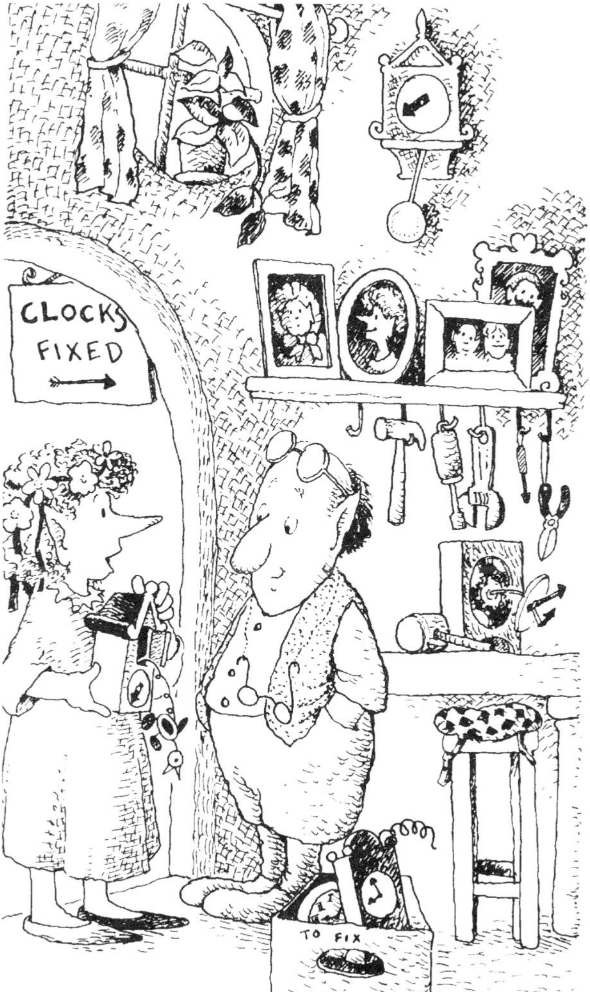
CLOCKS
FIXED
TO FIX

16.

The Golden Rule applies at your workplace: Treat your co-workers and your customers as you would like to be treated. The spirit that's created will enhance your work life and the lives of others.

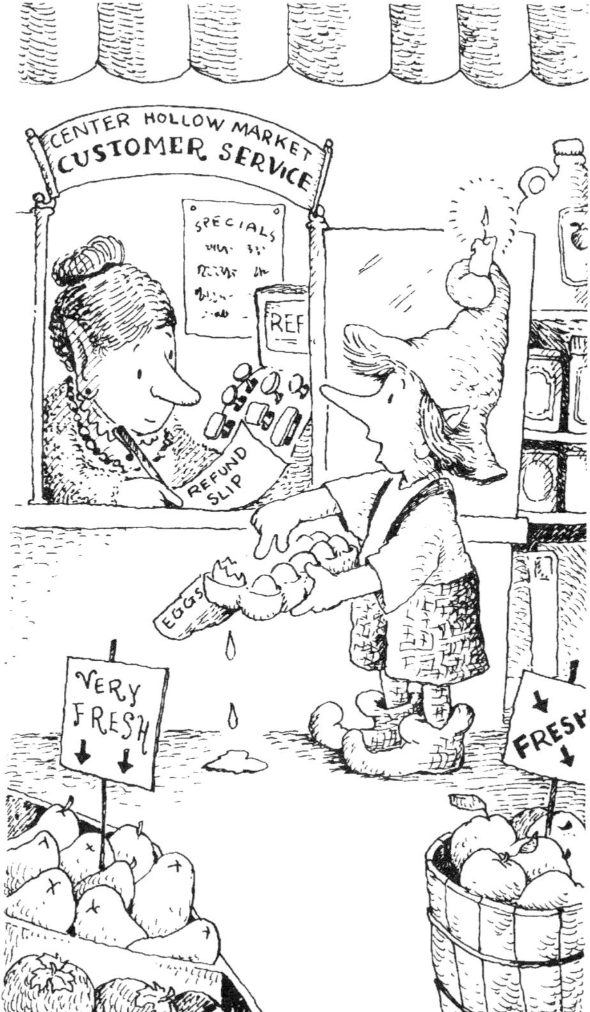
CENTER HOLLOW MARKET
CUSTOMER SERVICE
SPECIALS
REF
REFUND SLIP
EGGS
VERY FRESH
FRESH

17.

Work out conflicts on the job with charity, grace, and wisdom. Remember that the truth has many facets. Reach out in creative ways to help resolve disputes.

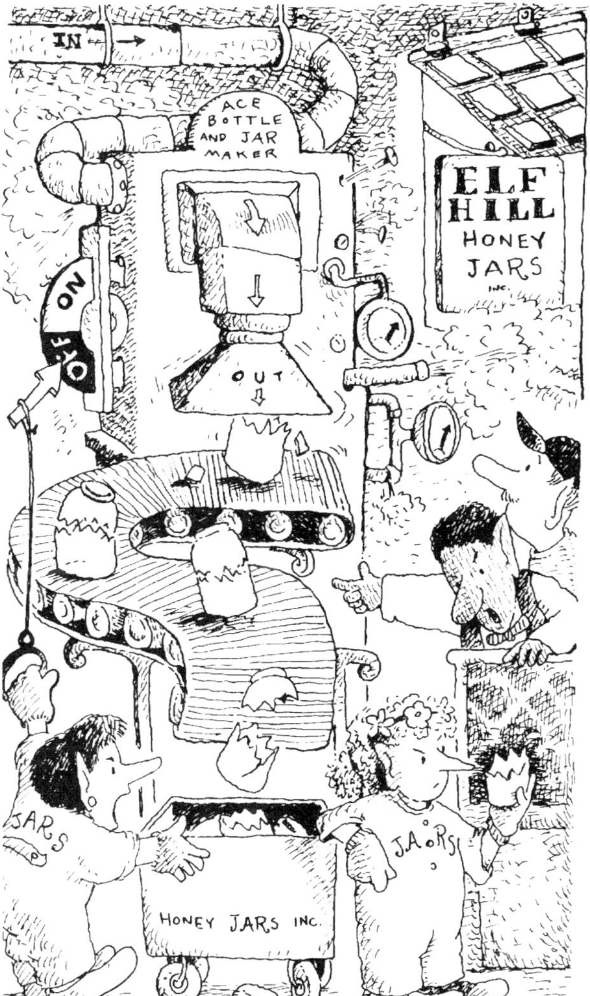
IN
ACE BOTTLE AND JAR MAKER
ON
OFF
OUT
ELF HILL HONEY JARS INC.
JARS
JARS
HONEY JARS INC.

18.

If something is broken, don't wait for someone else to fix it. Chip in and use your own unique skills and talents to make things better.

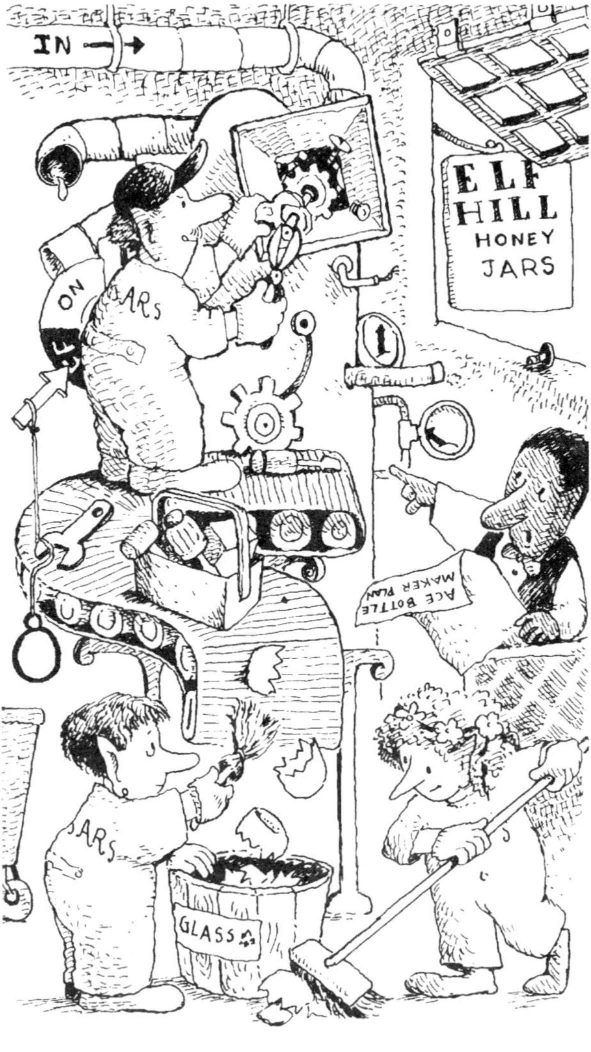
IN
ON
ELF
HILL
HONEY
JARS
ACE BOTTLE
MAKER PLAN
GLASS

19.

Every job has its less-than-perfect qualities, its difficult and discouraging periods. Make a list of all the good things about your work; refer to it on bad days.

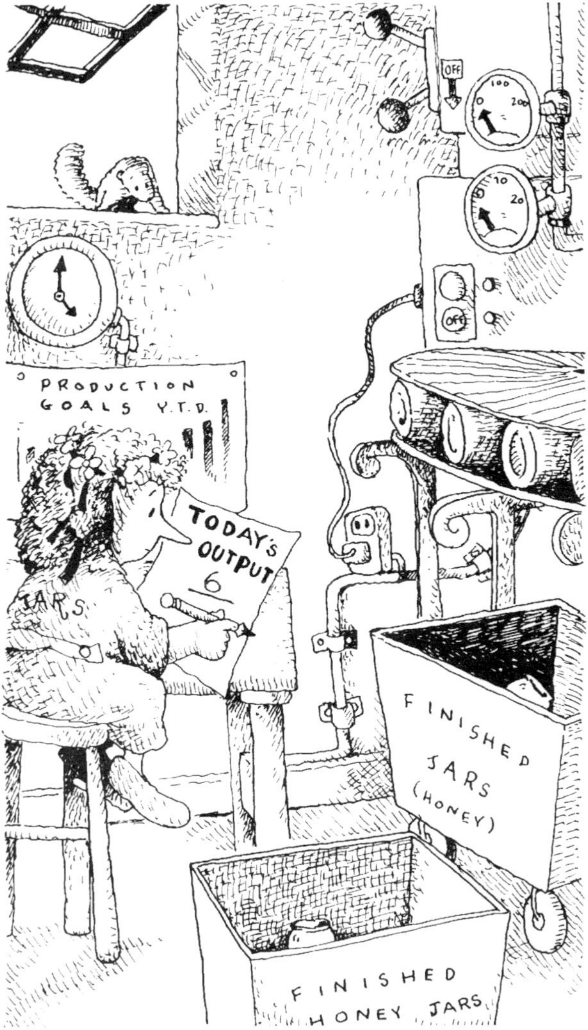
OFF
PRODUCTION GOALS Y.T.D.
TODAY'S OUTPUT 6
JARS
OFF
FINISHED JARS (HONEY)
FINISHED HONEY JARS

20.

If you're thinking about leaving a position or applying for a transfer, list the pluses and minuses of staying and of leaving. Weigh them thoughtfully and over time. Avoid rash decisions.

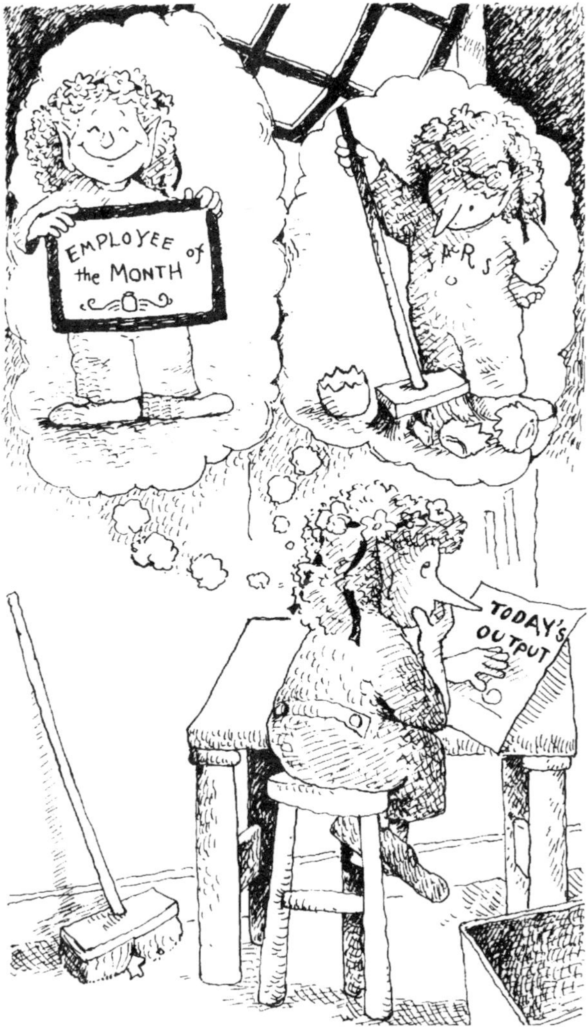
EMPLOYEE of the MONTH
TODAY'S OUTPUT

21.

If you're consistently unhappy with your work, if you never look forward to your workday, decide what would make you happy. Search for ways to make that dream real.

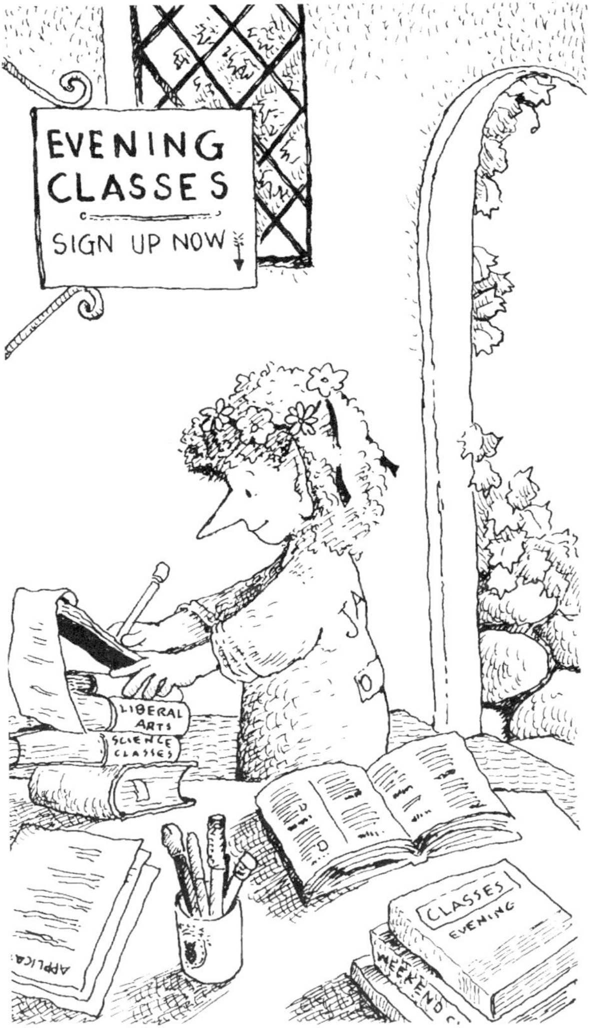
EVENING CLASSES
SIGN UP NOW
LIBERAL ARTS
SCIENCE CLASSES
CLASSES
EVENING
WEEKEND
APPLICA

22.

If you decide it's time to move on, leave on good terms. Don't burn any bridges. Leaving a job doesn't have to mean leaving good friends. Stay in touch.

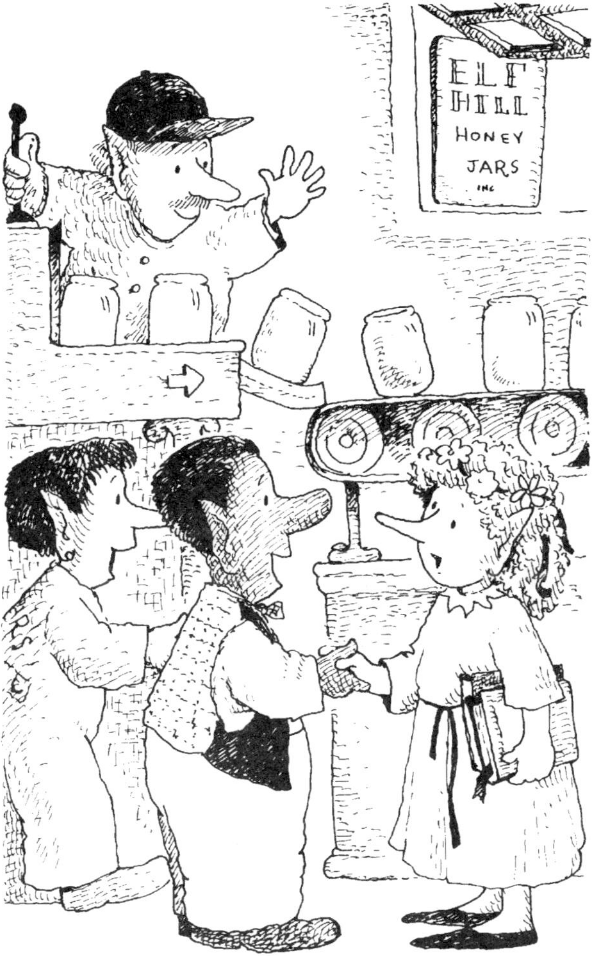
ELF
HILL
HONEY
JARS
INC

23.

Exploitation, harassment, and unjust working conditions do exist. If you feel you're being abused in your work setting, seek advice. Know your rights under the law.

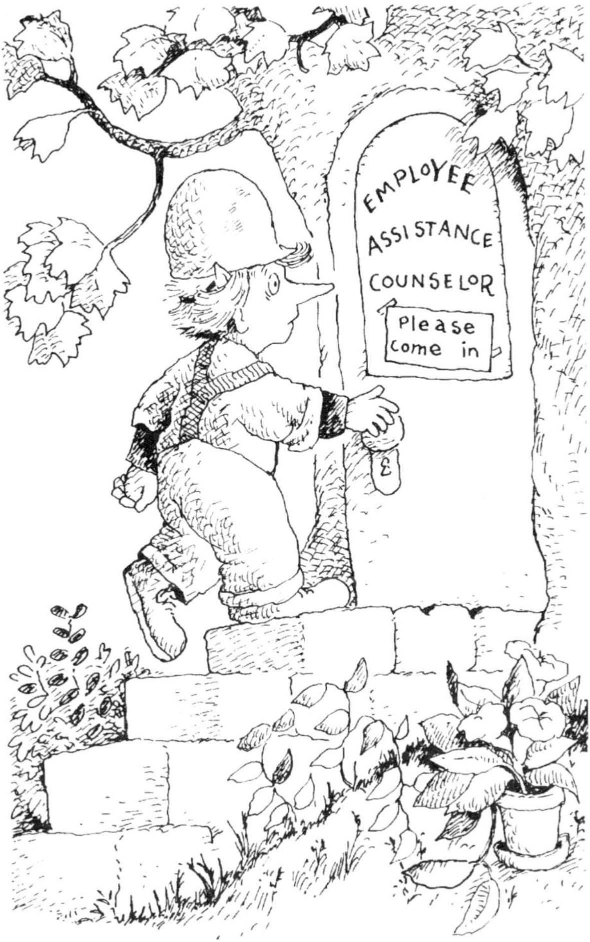
EMPLOYEE
ASSISTANCE
COUNSELOR
Please come in

24.

If you lose your job, don't lose faith in yourself. You are more than your job, and your worth is more than a paycheck.

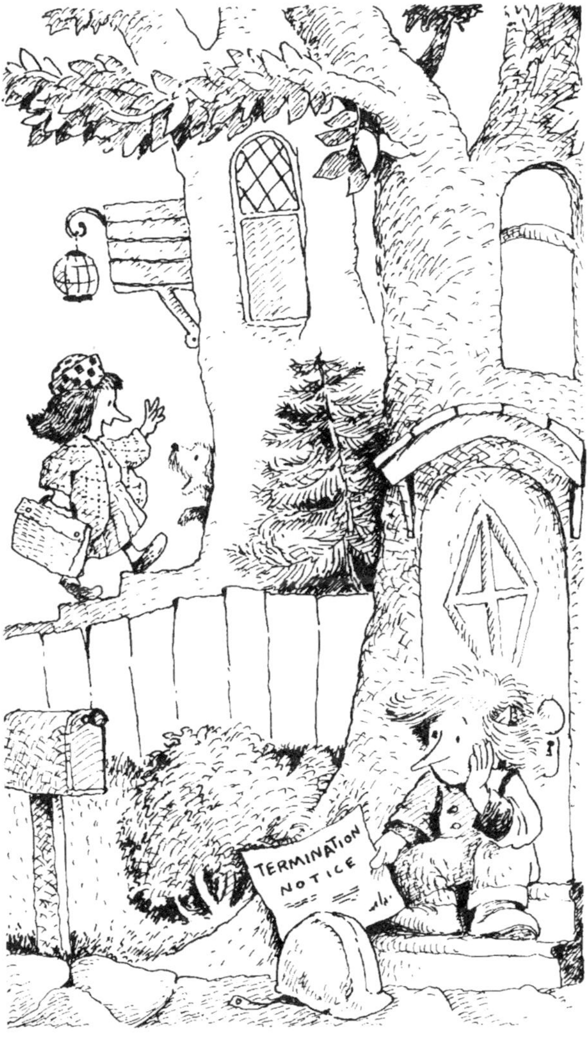
TERMINATION NOTICE

25.

When you lose a job or a hoped-for promotion, let yourself grieve, as you would for any other significant loss. Find healthy ways to express the pain and disappointment; then move on with your life.

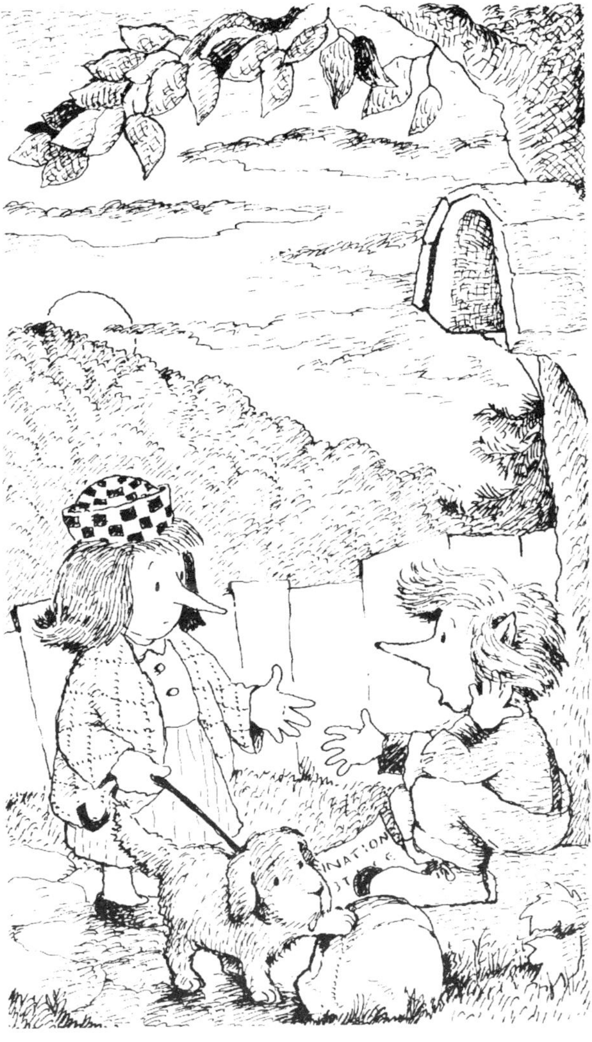

26.

When you're looking for work, make use of all available resources: friends, agencies, libraries, classified ads, the phone book. Treat the process of looking for a full-time job as a full-time job. It is.

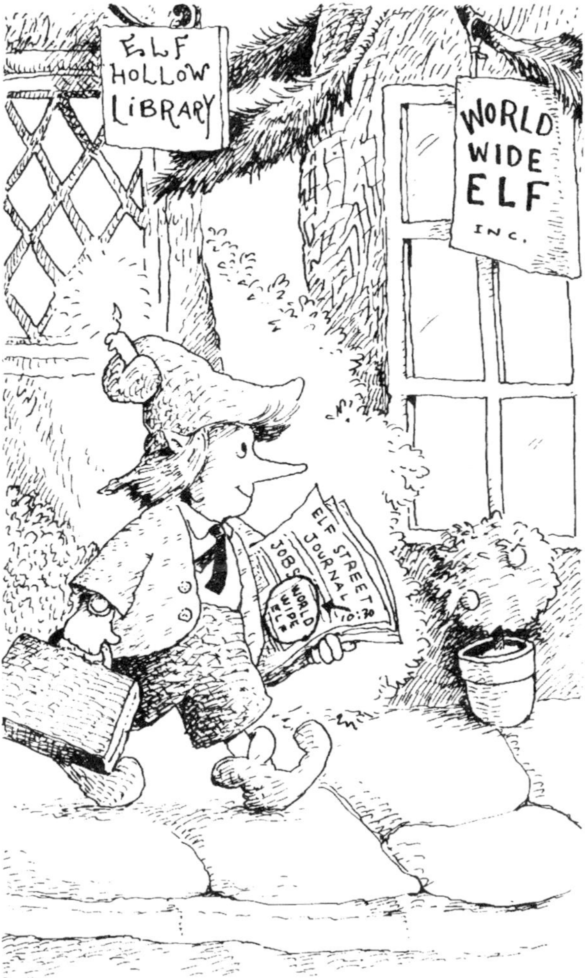
ELF HOLLOW LIBRARY
WORLD WIDE ELF INC.
ELF STREET JOURNAL
JOBS
WORLD WIPE ELF
10:30

27.

You may feel discouraged and anxious when you're unemployed. That's understandable. Find a sympathetic ear and share your feelings. Keep moving toward your goal. Cultivate patience and perseverance.

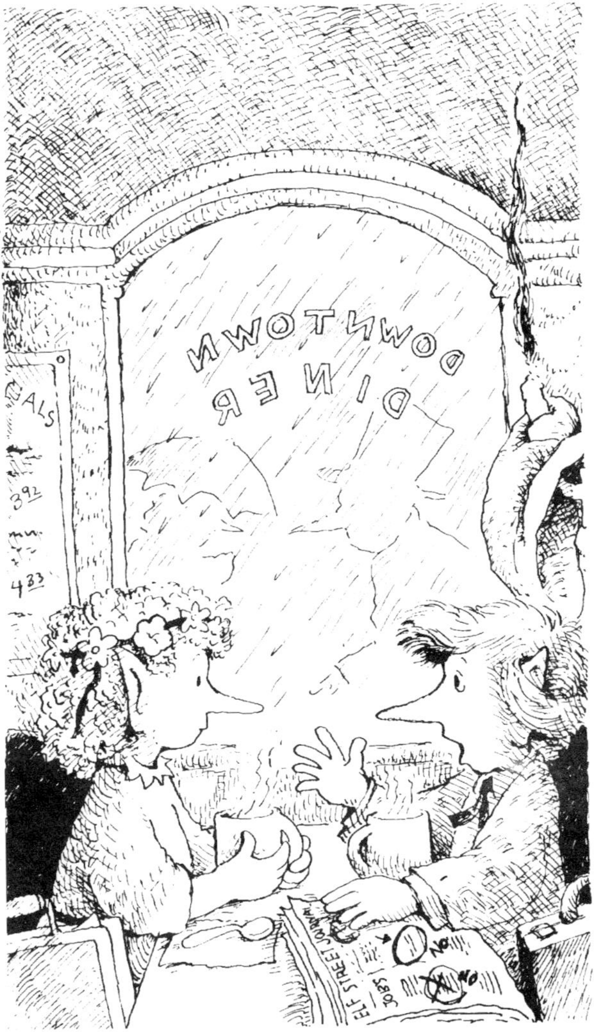
DOWNTOWN DINER
ALS
392
483
ELF STREET JOURNAL
JOBS
NO
NO

28.

When you're exploring new job possibilities, identify the skills and accomplishments you've attained over a lifetime of living. For instance, if you've raised a family, you've probably developed considerable abilities that would be valuable to an employer.

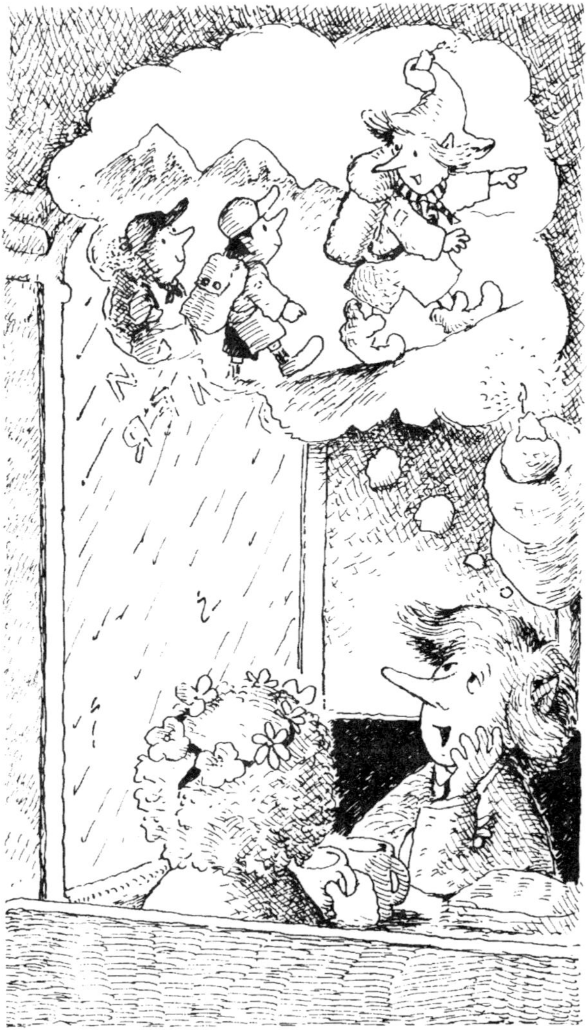

29.

The loss of a job can be an opportunity for learning, growth, change, and a new self-definition. Take stock of your gifts and pay attention to what your heart is telling you.

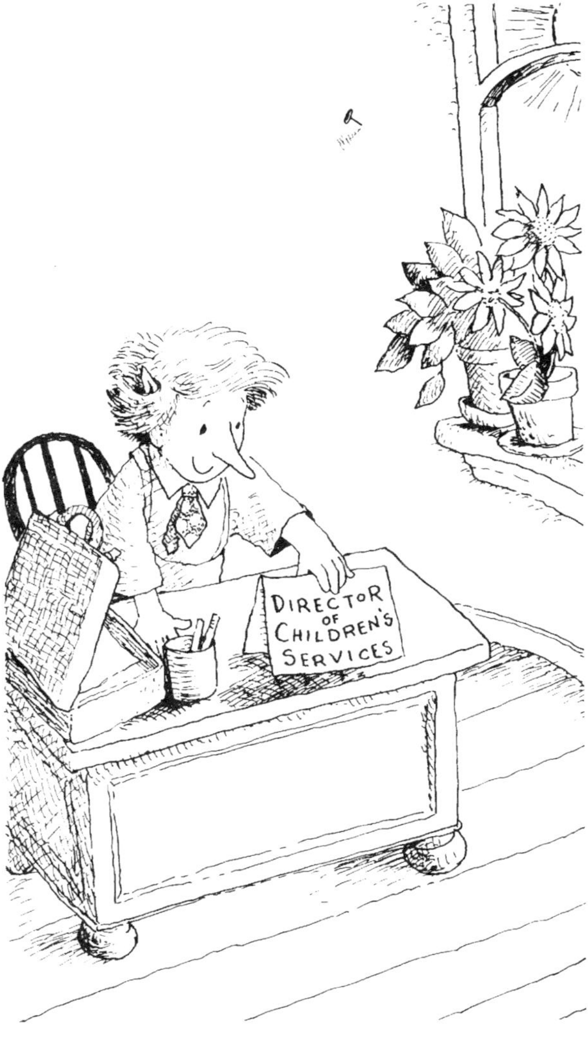
DIRECTOR
OF
CHILDREN'S
SERVICES

30.

Cultivate outside interests so that your life is more than your job. If you've forgotten how to play, spend time with children—or the child within you.

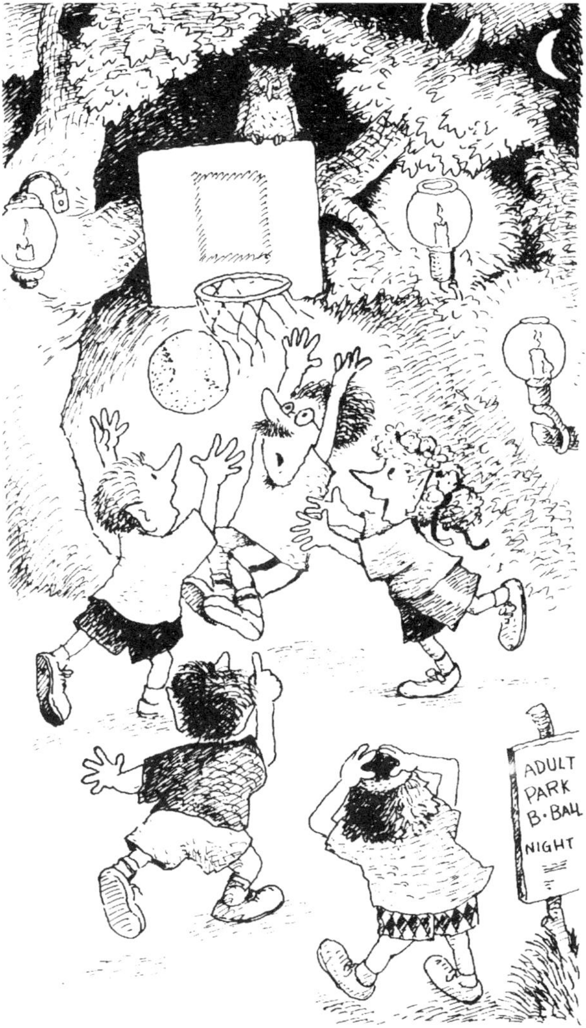
ADULT
PARK
B·BALL
NIGHT

31.

Volunteer work not only blesses those who receive it; it's a great source of satisfaction and growth for those who give it. Find a way to lend a hand and make your corner of the world a better place.

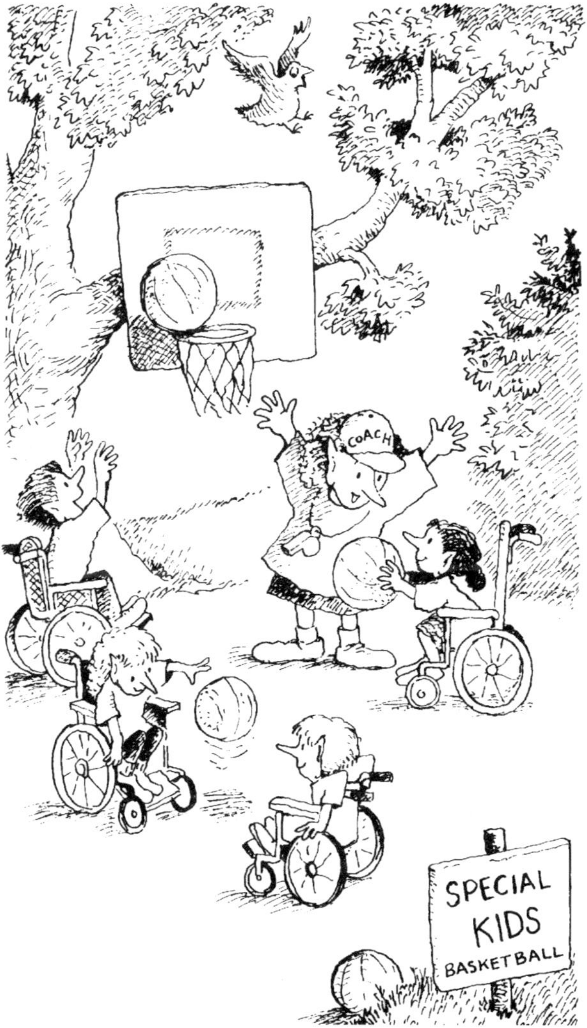
COACH
SPECIAL
KIDS
BASKETBALL

32.

If you sometimes need to take work home with you, do so intentionally. Other times, you may want to stay late and set boundaries to your workday. If you make conscious decisions about your work, you'll be more energized and focused.

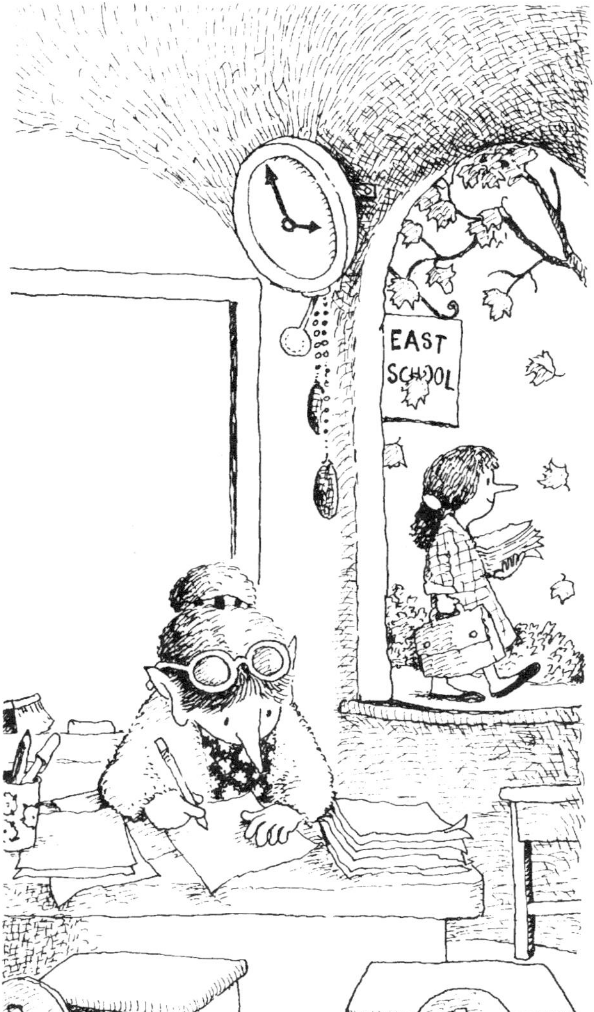
EAST
SCHOOL

33.

Don't work seven days a week. Your body, mind, and spirit need rest and renewal for you to be fully engaged in life. Even God took a day off.

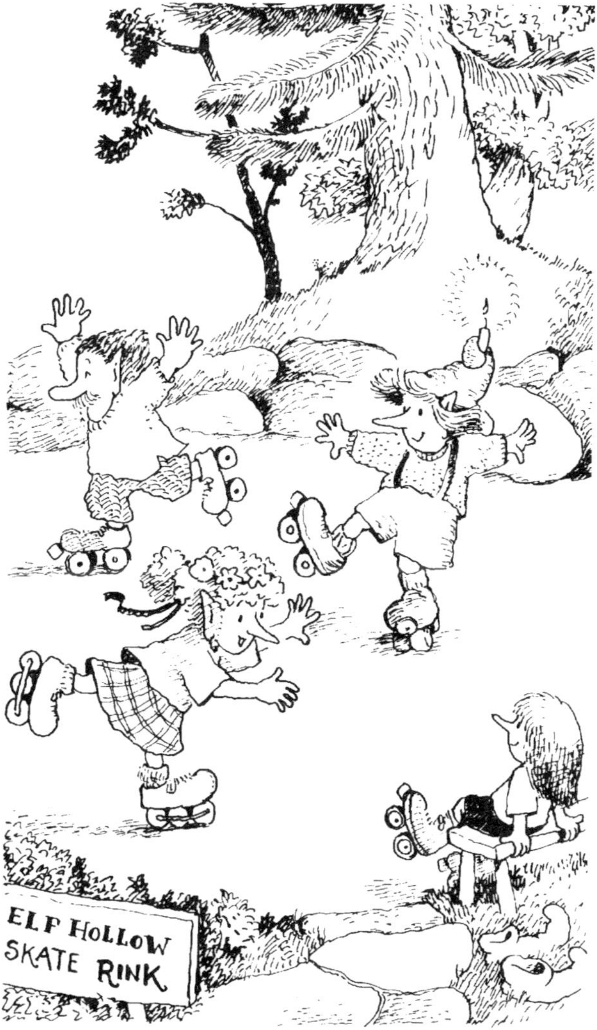
ELF HOLLOW
SKATE RINK

34.

When you go on vacation, really go on vacation. Don't drag your work with you, and don't assume "they can't get along" without you. They can. They will. Let them.

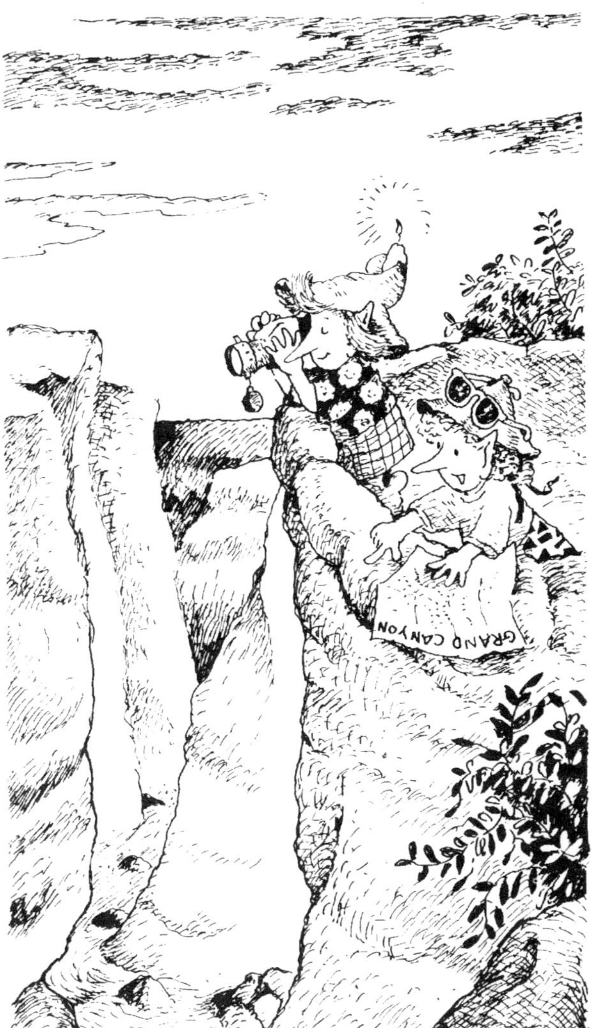
GRAND CANYON

35.

Fill in the blank: "At the end of my life, I will wish I had spent more time _____." Make this a reality now.

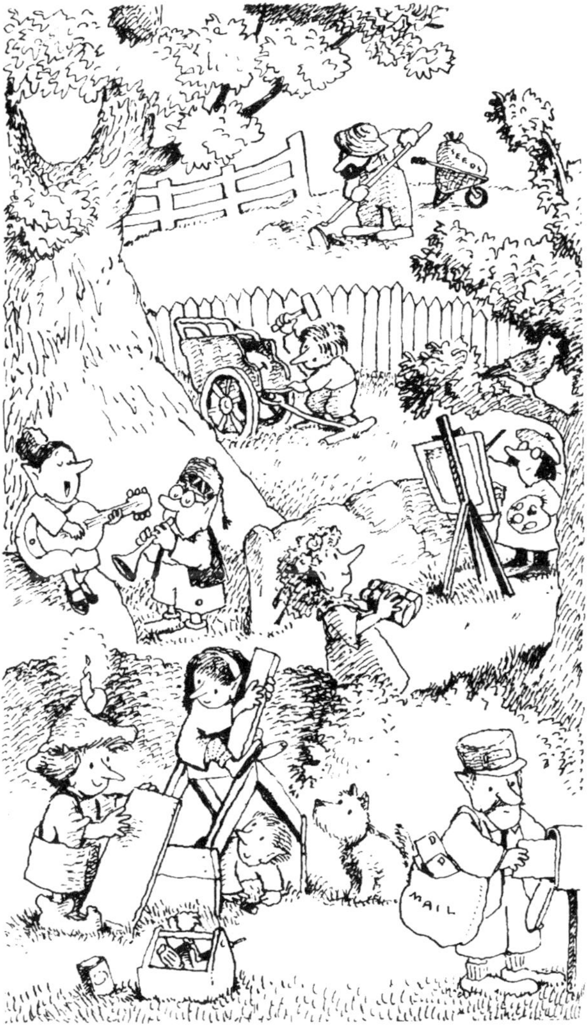
SEEDS
MAIL

An educator, author, and editor, **Daniel Grippo** lives in Prairie Village, Kansas. He says that he's "working on following the advice in *Work Therapy*."

Illustrator for the Abbey Press Elf-help Books, **R.W. Alley** also illustrates and writes children's books. He lives in Barrington, Rhode Island, with his wife, daughter, and son.

The Story of the Abbey Press Elves

The engaging figures that populate the Abbey Press "elf-help" line of publications and products first appeared in 1987 on the pages of a small self-help book called *Be-good-to-yourself Therapy*. Shaped by the publishing staff's vision and defined in R.W. Alley's inventive illustrations, they lived out author Cherry Hartman's gentle, self-nurturing advice with charm, poignancy, and humor.

Reader response was so enthusiastic that more Elf-help Books were soon under way, a still-growing series that has inspired a line of related gift products.

The especially endearing character featured in the early books—sporting a cap with a mood-changing candle in its peak—has since been joined by a spirited female elf with flowers in her hair.

These two exuberant, sensitive, resourceful, kindhearted, lovable sprites, along with their lively elfin community, reveal what's truly important as they offer messages of joy and wonder, playfulness and co-creation, wholeness and serenity, the miracle of life and the mystery of God's love.

With wisdom and whimsy, these little creatures with long noses demonstrate the elf-help way to a rich and fulfilling life.

Elf-help Books...adding "a little character" and a lot of help to self-help reading!

Work Therapy
#20166-5 $3.95 ISBN 0-87029-276-5

Everyday-courage Therapy
#20167-1 $3.95 ISBN 0-87029-274-9

Peace Therapy
#20176-4 $3.95 ISBN 0-87029-273-0

Friendship Therapy
#20174-9 $3.95 ISBN 0-87029-270-6

Christmas Therapy (color edition)
#20175-6 $5.95 ISBN 0-87029-268-4

Grief Therapy
#20178-0 $3.95 ISBN 0-87029-267-6

More Be-good-to-yourself Therapy
#20180-6 $3.95 ISBN 0-87029-262-5

Happy Birthday Therapy
#20181-4 $3.95 ISBN 0-87029-260-9

Forgiveness Therapy
#20184-8 $3.95 ISBN 0-87029-258-7

Keep-life-simple Therapy
#20185-5 $3.95 ISBN 0-87029-257-9

Be-good-to-your-body Therapy
#20188-9 $3.95 ISBN 0-87029-255-2

Celebrate-your-womanhood Therapy
#20189-7 $3.95 ISBN 0-87029-254-4

Acceptance Therapy (color edition)
#20182-2 $5.95 ISBN 0-87029-259-5

Acceptance Therapy (regular edition)
#20190-5 $3.95 ISBN 0-87029-245-5

Keeping-up-your-spirits Therapy
#20195-4 $3.95 ISBN 0-87029-242-0

Play Therapy
#20200-2 $3.95 ISBN 0-87029-233-1

Slow-down Therapy
#20203-6 $3.95 ISBN 0-87029-229-3

One-day-at-a-time Therapy
#20204-4 $3.95 ISBN 0-87029-228-5

Prayer Therapy
#20206-9 $3.95 ISBN 0-87029-225-0

Be-good-to-your-marriage Therapy
#20205-1 $3.95 ISBN 0-87029-224-2

Be-good-to-yourself Therapy (hardcover)
#20196-2 $10.95 ISBN 0-87029-243-9

Be-good-to-yourself Therapy
#20255-6 $3.95 ISBN 0-87029-209-9